ESSENTIAL GUIDE TO LICHEN PLANUS

Comprehensive Insights for Diagnosis, Treatment, and Management

DR. CASEY LOREN

DISCLAIMER

This book's content is only meant to be used for general informative purposes. Although the author has taken great care to ensure the content is accurate and thorough, no warranties or assurances on the information's accuracy, correctness, or reliability are provided. It is recommended that readers employ their own judgment and discretion when applying any material found in this book to their particular situation.

The information in this book is not intended to replace professional advice, nor is the author an expert in any of the subjects covered. It is recommended that readers consult with experienced professionals regarding any particular issues or concerns.

Any name that may be mentioned or referred in this book does not imply endorsement, recommendation, or relationship on the part of the author with any person, entity, good, website, or association. These references are made only for informational purposes and are not meant to be taken as recommendations or endorsements.

The information contained in this book may cause readers to suffer loss or damage, for which the author disclaims all obligation and accountability. The only people accountable for the decisions and actions taken by readers using the information presented are themselves.

Any names, characters, companies, locations, activities, occasions, and incidents referenced in this book are either made up or the result of the author's imagination. Any likeness to real people, living or dead, or to real things is entirely coincidental.

This book's content may change at any time, without prior notice, according to the author.

The onus is on the reader to verify whether there have been any updates or revisions.

The reader accepts the conditions of this disclaimer by reading this book. Please do not read this book or use its contents if you do not agree to these terms.

Table of Contents

CHAPTER 1

A BRIEF OVERVIEW OF ACNE

Lichen Planus Summary

An inflammatory skin ailment known as lichen planus can spread to other areas of the body, including the nails, genitalia, mouth, and skin. Itchy or painful little bumps with a flat top might appear on the skin or mucous membranes; this is the hallmark of this condition. An aberrant immune response is thought to be the actual cause of lichen planus, however, this is yet not completely understood.

The past and the present:

The medical literature initially documented lichen planus in the late 1800s. The mechanism and clinical signs of this condition have been better understood by researchers over the years.

Recent developments in immunology and dermatology have helped to clarify the pathophysiology of this illness, opening the door to more effective methods of diagnosis and treatment.

How Common Is Lichen Planus**

Although it is more frequent in adults, lichen planus can impact anyone of any age, race, or gender. Some people may be more likely to acquire lichen planus because of factors like heredity, autoimmune diseases, infections, or certain drugs. It should be noted, nevertheless, that not all individuals who possess these risk factors will develop the illness.

Lichen Planus Varieties and Types

Different types of lichen planus manifest in different ways and affect different parts of the body. There are a few different types of lichen planus, and they can manifest in different ways. One kind affects the skin, while another affects the mouth and oral mucosa. A fourth type affects the nails, while a fifth type affects the genital area. Each variation may manifest with unique symptoms and necessitate individualized treatment plans.

Myths That People Often Hold

A prevalent but false belief regarding lichen planus is that it can spread from person to person. Because it is not an infectious disease, lichen planus cannot spread from one individual to another. The idea that HPV can only affect the skin is another common misunderstanding since it can also affect other parts of the body, including the mucous membranes.

How It Affects People's Quality of Life:

The quality of life for those living with lichen planus might be greatly affected. Discomforting and interfering with day-to-day functioning, symptoms may include itching, discomfort, and changes in appearance. The possibility of a recurrence and the fact that the illness is chronic both add to the mental and emotional toll.

The Value of Being Informed

Early diagnosis, effective treatment, and support for lichen planus patients can only be achieved if the condition is better understood. It is important for healthcare providers, patients, and the public at large to be aware of the symptoms, indicators, and resources related to lichen planus.

The Purpose of This Manual

This guide aims to serve as a thorough resource for anybody interested in lichen planus. It covers all the bases, from epidemiology to clinical aspects, diagnosis to treatment choices, and even coping mechanisms. We hope that by covering these bases, people will be better able to comprehend and control lichen planus.

Use of This Book Instructions

The book is structured in a way that readers can easily find the sections they're interested in, as they address different elements of lichen planus. With the use of helpful graphics, case studies, and advice, readers will be able to better grasp the material and make educated decisions.

The skin, mucous membranes, nails, and genitalia can all be affected by lichen planus, an inflammatory disorder that lasts for a long time.

It has been the subject of substantial research since its description in the late 1800s.

Lichen planus can affect anyone, however, some things might make it more likely.

Skin, mouth, nail, and vaginal lichen planus variants are all possible.

Its limited impact and infectiousness are two common misunderstandings.

It's important to be aware of lichen planus and provide support because it can have a substantial impact on quality of life.

Those who suffer from lichen planus might find information and strength in this guide.

CHAPTER 2

POSSIBLE ROOTS AND DANGERS

Knowing How the Immune System Works:

An immune-mediated condition, lichen planus occurs when the body's immune system attacks its tissues. Lichen planus is characterized by inflammation and the development of distinctive lesions that occur when T cells—a kind of white blood cell—attack the skin or mucous membranes. To create treatments that target immunological pathways, it is essential to understand this immune response.

Predisposition in the Family Tree:

There is some evidence that lichen planus is hereditary, however it is not the only cause. When exposed to environmental triggers or infections, some people may have a higher risk of acquiring lichen planus due to certain genetic differences. Nevertheless, additional studies are required to gain a complete understanding of the hereditary aspect of lichen planus.

Factors Influencing the Environment:

Several environmental variables have the potential to cause or worsen lichen planus. Chemicals, allergens, or even skin or mucous membrane injuries can fall into this category. To better manage the illness and lessen the frequency of flare-ups, it is helpful to identify and prevent certain triggers.

Lichen Planus Caused by Medications

As a side effect, lichen planus can be triggered by some drugs. Certain antibiotics, NSAIDs, and medications for hypertension and cardiovascular disease may fall into this category. When providing drugs to patients, healthcare providers must be mindful of these potential relationships.

Infections and Their Role:

Lichen planus has been associated with illnesses, especially viral ones like hepatitis C. One theory suggests that autoimmune reactions to certain infections can play a role in the onset of lichen planus lesions. To effectively manage lichen planus, it is crucial to address any underlying infections that may be present.

The Role of Hormones

The onset or worsening of lichen planus may be influenced by hormonal changes, like those that happen during pregnancy or menopause. Interactions between the immune system and hormones may be at the heart of the currently unexplained processes underlying these hormonal effects.

Psychological and Stress-Related Considerations:

Lichen planus can be influenced by stress and psychological variables. Although stress may not be the direct cause of lichen planus, it can worsen the symptoms or produce flare-ups when they already exist. People with lichen planus may find better results if they learn to manage their stress through counseling, relaxation techniques, or other interventions.

Coexisting Illnesses

Some medical illnesses, such as autoimmune diseases (like lupus), liver ailments (like hepatitis), and metabolic disorders (like diabetes), have been linked to lichen planus. For all-encompassing patient care, including treatment methods, understanding these relationships is crucial.

Demographic Risk Factors:

Although lichen planus can strike at any age or among any demography, it may be more common in some populations. For instance, it may manifest differently depending on race or geographical region, and it disproportionately affects middle-aged adults. Early diagnosis and management can be facilitated by identifying these demographic risk factors.

Recent Findings from the Field:

New information about lichen planus is being uncovered by researchers all the time. This includes possible diagnostic biomarkers, new therapy targets, and genetic predispositions. Researchers, clinicians, and patients are working together to better understand this complex disorder and achieve better patient outcomes.

Healthcare professionals can enhance patient outcomes by gaining a greater understanding of lichen planus and its facets, which in turn allows for more personalized treatment plans.

CHAPTER 3

SIGNS AND EVALUATION

What You Can Expect From Lichen Planus

Signs and symptoms of lichen planus may manifest on the skin and in the mucous membranes. Some of the most prevalent symptoms are:

1. **Lesions on the Skin**: These are reddish-purple papules that are flat-topped and glossy. Fine white streaks, known as Wickham's striae, may be present in certain lesions.

2. Itching, also known as pruritus, is a common symptom of skin lesions and can be quite uncomfortable, ranging from mild to severe.

3. **Involvement of the Mucosa**: The erosive type of lichen planus causes open sores, whereas the reticular pattern causes white, lacy

patches on the mucous membranes lining the mouth and genitalia, among other places.

4. **Changes to the Nails**: On extremely rare occasions, lichen planus can cause the nails to become thinner, develop ridges or grooves, or even undergo dystrophy.

5. **Scalp Involvement**: Redness, scaling, and hair loss (lichen planopilaris) can occur when lichen planus affects the scalp.

Oral Lichen Planus: How to Spot It

The interior mucosa of the mouth is the most common target of oral lichen planus. It might manifest as open sores (erosive form) or white, lacy patches (reticular form) on the palate, gums, tongue, and cheeks. Pain, burning, or sensitivity to spicy or hot meals are all possible side effects for patients.

The appearance of flat-topped, glossy, reddish-purple papules on the genitalia, lower back, ankles, and wrists is a hallmark of cutaneous lichen planus. Itching could be a symptom, and things like stress and some drugs might make it worse.

Involvement of the Nails and Scalps

Alterations including ridges, grooves, weakening, or even loss of nails can result from lichen planus's involvement with the nails. The symptoms of lichen planopilaris, which affects the scalp, include redness, scaling, and thinning hair.

Possible Diagnosis

It is critical to be able to differentiate lichen planus from other skin disorders. Fungal infections, allergic responses, psoriasis, eczema, and lupus erythematosus are among the possible differential diagnoses. Correct diagnosis requires comprehensive diagnostic testing in addition to a comprehensive clinical evaluation.

Criteria for Diagnosis

The hallmark lesions and mucosal involvement make lichen planus a clinically significant diagnosis. To rule out other comparable disorders, you need to have polygonal papules with Wickham's striae, mucosal involvement, and a lack of other symptoms.

The Diagnostic Importance of Biopsy

To confirm the diagnosis of lichen planus, a biopsy of the skin or mucosa may be taken. Characteristic alterations in the dermis and epidermis, as well as apoptotic keratinocytes (Civatte bodies) and a lymphocytic infiltration shaped like a band, are shown by histopathological investigation.

The Function of Laboratory Tests

When trying to diagnose a health problem or rule out alternative possibilities, laboratory testing can be quite helpful. Hepatitis screening, liver function tests, and complete blood counts (CBCs) may be ordered if the doctor suspects hepatitis C, which is often associated with lichen planus.

Radiological Exams

Skin lesion evaluation and progression tracking may be aided by imaging studies like dermoscopy. Unless other problems, such as squamous cell carcinoma, are detected, imaging is usually not necessary to diagnose lichen planus.

The Exam and Patient History

Medications, allergies, family history of autoimmune diseases, when symptoms first appeared, and the length of time the patient has been experiencing them should all be part of a thorough patient history. Lichen planus can be diagnosed with a comprehensive physical examination that includes the scalp, nails, skin, and mucous membranes.

Finally, skin and mucosal symptoms of lichen planus are unique, necessitating a thorough evaluation, diagnostic testing, and differential diagnosis for correct diagnosis and treatment.

CHAPTER 4

THE SCIENCE OF DISEASE AND ITS CAUSES

Lichen Planus and the Immune Response

Inflammation is the main symptom of lichen planus, skin, and mucous membrane disorder. Investigating the complex relationship between immune responses, cellular processes, and molecular pathways is essential for comprehending its pathophysiology and disease etiology.

Mechanisms at the Cellular and Molecular Levels

Lichen planus activates immune cells, especially T lymphocytes, on a cellular level. The inflammatory mediators chemokines and cytokines are released when these cells penetrate the injured tissues. Cell signaling pathways, such as those involved in inflammation and apoptosis (programmed cell death), change the condition.

The Function of T-Cells

In the pathophysiology of lichen planus, T-cells are pivotal. They detect antigens and react by starting an immune cascade after being attracted to the site of inflammation. One feature of lichen planus is an imbalance in the subsets of T-cells, which leads to tissue destruction. This imbalance is most pronounced in the CD8+ cytotoxic T-cell subset.

Presentation of Antigens and Activation of the Immune System

An essential part of activating the immune system is the presentation of antigens, usually via dendritic cells. Lichen planus is caused by the activation and inflammation of T-cells in response to antigens that might originate from either the body or the environment. A dysregulation of this mechanism, as shown in autoimmune diseases like lichen planus, can occur.

Routes of Inflammation

Several mechanisms, such as the NF-κB pathway and the JAK-STAT pathway, are involved in the orchestration of inflammation in lichen planus. Tissue damage and clinical symptoms are influenced by these pathways, which control the expression of chemokines, pro-inflammatory cytokines, and adhesion molecules.

Disease Chronology and Persistence

Chronic lichen planus is a common skin condition that can last for a long time. The disease's chronicity is caused by the ongoing activation of immunological responses, which in turn cause tissue destruction and remodeling. Disease persistence can be influenced by factors like genetic predisposition and environmental triggers.

Effects on the Dermis and Lungs

In addition to the skin, genitalia, the oral cavity, and the gastrointestinal system are also mucosal membranes that can be affected by lichen planus. The distinctive lesions, which include papules, plaques, and erosions, can lead to pain, discomfort, and impaired functionality, greatly affecting the quality of life for those afflicted.

The possibility of cancerous transformation

The possibility of malignant transformation is a major worry with lichen planus, especially in mucosal forms like oral lichen planus. Dysplasia and squamous cell carcinoma are more likely to develop in conditions of chronic inflammation and tissue injury. To effectively manage this risk, it is crucial to conduct regular monitoring and intervene early on.

Studying the Causes of Disease

Researchers are constantly trying to figure out what causes lichen planus and how it works. This includes research on environmental causes, genetic variables, molecular processes, and immune cell dysregulation. We are learning more about the disease thanks to technological advancements like genomic analysis and high-resolution imaging.

New Hypotheses and Theories

Microbiota dysbiosis, epigenetic alterations, and immune cell plasticity are some of the newer ideas and theories in lichen planus study. Future personalized and tailored treatments may be possible thanks to the fresh understanding of disease pathophysiology and possible therapeutic targets provided by these research areas.

In conclusion, environmental factors, immunological responses, cellular connections, and molecular pathways all play a role in the complicated inflammatory condition known as lichen planus. If we want to improve therapy efficacy and patient outcomes, we need to learn more about its pathogenesis.

CHAPTER 5

APPROACHES TO TREATMENT

Treatments Applied Topically

When treating localized lichen planus, topical treatments are typically the initial line of defense. Medication used topically to the skin or mucous membranes is a common component of these treatments. Topical corticosteroids are a common choice since they alleviate inflammation and irritation. It is possible to utilize non-steroidal alternatives, such as calcineurin inhibitors, in sensitive areas, such as the face or genitalia. Applying a moisturizer or emollient can help alleviate the dryness and pain caused by lichen planus lesions.

Medications Used Systemically

Medications Used Systemically

Systemic medicines may be recommended for lichen planus cases that are more extensive or severe. These drugs have a systemic effect and are typically administered intravenously or orally. Systemic administration of corticosteroids is an option for more severe or resistant patients. Systemic alternatives include immunomodulatory medicines such as methotrexate or cyclosporine, as well as retinoids, which aid in controlling cell proliferation and differentiation.

Treatment using light

Lichen planus lesions can be treated using phototherapy, which uses light of specified wavelengths. There is some evidence that therapy with ultraviolet (UV) light, specifically UVB and PUVA (psoralen plus UVA), helps alleviate inflammation and other symptoms. In situations where systemic drugs might not be an option or when previous therapies have failed, phototherapy is frequently considered.

Agents that weaken the immune system

Lichen planus is an autoimmune disorder in which the immune system assaults healthy tissues; immunosuppressive agents are medicines that reduce the activity of the immune system and may help with the treatment of this condition. Corticosteroids and other targeted immunosuppressants such as mycophenolate mofetil or azathioprine may be among these drugs. In addition to reducing inflammation, they help stop additional harm to the skin and mucous membranes.

Biotherapeutic Interventions

Biologic treatments are a relatively new kind of medicine that aims to modulate the immune system by influencing particular molecules. Although lichen planus has not been examined thoroughly, biologics such as interleukin inhibitors or TNF-alpha inhibitors may be useful in some cases when other treatments have failed to alleviate the condition sufficiently.

Healthcare Approaches Other Than Conventional Medicine

Patients who aren't getting enough relief from their current treatments may look into complementary and alternative medicine. Aloe vera, turmeric, acupuncture, homeopathy, vitamin D, and omega-3 fatty acid supplements are some examples of herbal therapies. It is important to proceed with caution when considering these treatments for lichen planus, even if they may be useful for some people.

Diet and Nutrition: Their Role

Although there is a lack of clear evidence about the efficacy of dietary interventions in the treatment of lichen planus, it is reasonable to assume that a healthy, balanced diet will have a positive effect on both the condition and general health. Certain meals or drinks, such as spicy cuisine or acidic drinks, may make some people's symptoms worse. Sometimes it helps to know what sets off such episodes so you can stay away from them. Supporting skin and mucosal health can also be achieved by consuming nutrient-rich foods and staying well-hydrated.

Changes to Your Way of Life

Making changes to one's way of life can have a big impact on controlling lichen planus. Reduce the frequency and severity of flare-ups by avoiding things that bring them on, like stress, particular drugs, or irritants. For oral lichen planus, it's crucial to practice proper oral hygiene, which includes seeing the dentist regularly and utilizing gentle oral care products. Excessive sun exposure and damage can worsen lesions, thus it's important to protect the skin.

Controlling Adverse Reactions

Side effects are a possibility with many lichen planus therapies, particularly systemic drugs. Healthcare personnel must attentively observe patients and swiftly address any negative reactions. Possible adverse effects should be communicated to patients and they should be urged to report any unexpected symptoms. To reduce the risk of side effects while keeping the medicine effective, it may be required to change the dosage or try an alternate therapy.

Responding to and Tracking Treatment

Managing lichen planus requires close observation of the patient's reaction to treatment. Symptom reduction, improvement in lesion appearance, and enhanced quality of life are some ways that healthcare providers can measure improvement. It is possible to modify treatment regimens as required with the help of regular follow-up visits. The effectiveness of treatment, the presence of side effects, or the rate of disease progression can all be assessed with further diagnostic procedures, such as biopsies.

CHAPTER 6

COPING WITH ECZEMA

A Skincare Programme for Every Day:

Those who suffer from lichen planus must adhere to a strict skincare regimen to alleviate symptoms and maintain healthy skin. To keep things from getting irritated, this regimen usually includes using moderate, fragrance-free soaps or cleansers for washing. Even more so with hypoallergenic goods free of possible allergens, moisturizing is essential. Another crucial factor is to shield yourself from the sun since lichen planus symptoms might worsen when exposed to UV rays. For that reason, it's advised to use a broad-spectrum sunscreen that has an SPF of 30 or above.

Keeping Your Teeth Healthy

Keeping Your Teeth Healthy

It is crucial to maintain good oral hygiene since lichen planus can potentially affect the mucosa of the mouth. This involves flossing regularly to remove plaque and using a soft-bristled toothbrush with fluoride toothpaste regularly. If you suffer from sensitive oral tissues, it may help to use a mouthwash that is free of alcohol and other harsh substances. Also, it's smart to get your teeth checked often so you can catch any abnormalities in your mouth cavity early and fix them before they worsen.

Living with Pain and Itching:

Lichen planus is characterized by itching and pain; however, there are ways to alleviate these symptoms. To alleviate itching, try using a cool compress, a mild moisturizer, or an over-the-counter anti-itch lotion with hydrocortisone or calamine. You can also lessen the itching and discomfort by staying away from things that make it worse, like hot showers, rough clothes, and spicy food.

Counseling and Psychological Support:

Mental health might suffer when dealing with a long-term illness like lichen planus. Counseling and psychological support can help with the emotional difficulties of living with the disease. Some people find that therapy helps with anxiety, despair, or the stress that comes with dealing with symptoms and making lifestyle changes.

Flare-Up Management:

It is critical to manage flare-ups, when lichen planus symptoms worsen, to maintain quality of life. One way to keep flare-ups at bay is to learn what sets them off, whether it's stress, particular meals, or environmental variables. To manage symptoms during flare-ups, a healthcare provider may prescribe oral or topical medicines.

Why It's Crucial to Check In Often

To keep an eye on lichen planus and make any necessary adjustments to treatment, it is crucial to have regular follow-up visits with healthcare specialists. At these checkups, we can assess how your symptoms are doing, make note of any problems, and figure out how to best manage your condition so that you have the best possible outcome and quality of life.

Resources and Support Groups:

You can find helpful information, emotional support, and a feeling of community by joining a support group or looking for internet resources that are specific to lichen planus. Frequently, these sites provide instructional materials, platforms for exchanging stories, and chances to meet people going through the same things you are.

Work and social life strategies:

Strategies for managing lichen planus in social and occupational contexts may include being upfront and honest with coworkers and employers about the condition and the modifications that may be required. You can also lessen the impact on your day-to-day life and social plans by preparing ahead of time for possible flare-ups or symptom exacerbations.

Personal Narratives and Experiences of Patients:

Reading about other people's experiences with lichen planus can provide comfort, understanding, and affirmation. Inspiration, coping mechanisms, and practical advice for dealing with the condition's difficulties can be found in patient experiences published through healthcare organizations, support groups, or blogs.

*Projection into the Future**

Despite the long-term nature of lichen planus, many people can control their symptoms and continue leading fulfilling lives with the help of medication and self-care. It's critical to communicate any worries or changes in symptoms quickly and collaborate closely with healthcare professionals to create a tailored management plan. People with lichen planus have a better chance of a healthy long-term prognosis if they assess their condition regularly and follow treatment recommendations.

CHAPTER 7

TARGET AUDIENCES

Primary Source on Lichen
Planus: Target Groups

Chronic inflammatory dermatitis (also known as lichen planus) can manifest on hair, nails, mucous membranes, and skin. To effectively manage and cure it, understanding how it affects different populations is essential. In this article, we go into the complexities of lichen planus in various age groups, genders, ethnicities, co-occurring diseases, immunocompromised individuals, patients, and their sexual health. For a full grasp, we also give case stories and talk about pediatric management tactics.

The Signs and Manifestations

Plaques and pruritic, violaceous papules with flat tops are indications of lichen planus, which is less frequent in children compared to adults. The lower back, ankles, and wrists are common sites for lesions to manifest in youngsters. Additionally, white, lacy patches might be visible in the mouth as a sign of oral involvement.

This is the diagnosis:

A skin biopsy may be necessary to confirm a clinical diagnosis of lichen planus in children and to rule out other possible causes, such as eczema, psoriasis, or viral exanthems.

Medical Approach

Topical corticosteroids are the usual treatment for inflammation and irritation in children. Systemic therapies including phototherapy, immunosuppressive drugs, or oral corticosteroids may be required in extreme instances. Encouraging patients to stick to their treatment plans requires both knowledge and assistance.

** Lichen Planus and Pregnancy**

Effects on the Unborn Child

The fetus is unaffected by lichen planus, however, the condition can make pregnancy more difficult. Nevertheless, the health of mothers might be affected by the pain and anxiety caused by symptoms.

Things to Think About When Treating

Prenatal care must strike a balance between the benefits to the mother and the risks to the unborn child. It is important to exercise caution and seek medical supervision when using systemic corticosteroids, however, topical corticosteroids are typically safe. Emollients and stress reduction strategies are non-pharmacological therapies that can also be helpful.

Care and Monitoring

To properly manage symptoms and maintain the health of both the mother and the fetus, pregnant women with lichen planus must undergo regular monitoring. Consult your obstetrician and dermatologist regularly for checkups.

Presenting and Overcoming Obstacles

Changes in the skin that come with getting older and a possible reduction in the immune response make the symptoms of lichen planus more noticeable in older people. Oral involvement is prevalent, and lesions might be more extensive.

Management Approaches

The possibility of comorbidities and polypharmacy should be taken into account when treating aged people. The use of topical corticosteroids is still common, but systemic treatments should be approached with caution to prevent unwanted side effects. It is crucial to prioritize mild skin care and stay away from anything that could irritate the skin.

It is essential to educate senior people on how to properly care for their skin, stick to their treatment plans, and deal with itching. Carers' encouragement can improve patients' adherence to therapy and their quality of life generally.

Presentational Disparities Based on Gender

Different Symptoms

Although lichen planus can impact either sex, research has shown that the two may manifest differently. Involvement in the mouth and genitalia is more common in women, whereas skin lesions may be more widespread in men.

Treatment Consequences

More personalized treatment approaches can be guided by understanding gender-specific symptoms. When it comes to vulvar discomfort and potential problems like adhesions, women with genital lichen planus may need specialized care.

Varieties in Lichen Planus Across Ethnic Groups

Occurrence and Display

various ethnic groups may experience lichen planus at various rates and in diverse ways. Hyperpigmentation after lichen planus, for example, is more common among people of color, which can have an impact on both the aesthetic results and the psychological and social health of those affected.

Approaches to Treatment

Different ethnic groups need different approaches to therapy. Topical retinoids or hydroquinone, for instance, might be used alongside conventional therapies to relieve post-inflammatory hyperpigmentation. Managing patients from varied backgrounds requires cultural awareness and empathy.

Conditions That Occur Together

The Most Common Illnesses

Hepatitis C, diabetes, and autoimmune illnesses are common co-occurring ailments with lichen planus. It is crucial to acknowledge these connections to provide thorough patient care.

Efficient Management System

It is important to screen for and treat any co-occurring diseases as part of the management process. Antiviral treatment for hepatitis C, for example, may alleviate lichen planus symptoms in certain patients.

Treatment for Patients with Reduced Immunity Function

The Difficulties

Lichen planus can be more severe and difficult to treat in immunocompromised patients, such as those dealing with HIV/AIDS or going through chemotherapy. Treatment complications and increased infection risk may result from their immunological state.

Things to Think About When Treating

Minimizing immunosuppression should be the goal of treatments. While topical therapies are usually the best option, systemic medications such as acitretin or low-dose methotrexate may be tried under close medical supervision.

Working together with the patient's primary care physician or oncologist is frequently essential.

Effects on Family Planning

Genital Eczema

When lichen planus spreads to the vaginal regions, it can cause a great deal of pain, suffering, and even infertility. Vulvar erosions in women and penile lesions in men are possible.

Making a Difference in Sexual Health

Sexual health should be a topic of open discussion. Immunosuppressants, topical steroids, and pain management techniques are among the possible treatments. When dealing with the psychological and social effects, it may be helpful to see a psychologist or a sexual health expert.

Pediatric Care Approaches

Customized Methods

Lichen planus in children needs to be managed using strategies that are suitable for their age. After weighing the benefits and risks, topical corticosteroids are typically administered as a first line of defense.

Help with Learning and Support

Family education regarding the disease's chronicity, treatment adherence, and lifestyle changes is crucial. The family and the child can benefit emotionally from attending a support group or seeing a counselor.

Examples and Case Studies

Examples of Illustrations

1. Case Study 1: A Youth Suffering with Cutaneous Lichen Planus

A 7-year-old boy presents with painful, purple papules on his ankles and wrists.

The diagnosis of lichen planus was made after a thorough clinical examination and a biopsy.

- Antihistamines and topical corticosteroids are used to treat itching. Significant improvement was observed with regular follow-ups.

2. **Second Case Study: A Woman's Experience with Oral Lichen Planus**

The patient is a 32-year-old pregnant woman who presents with sores in her mouth.

- Oral examination and biopsy for diagnosis.

- Oral hygiene measures and topical corticosteroids are used as treatments. No detrimental effects on pregnancy were observed due to regular monitoring.

3. **Severe Lichen Planus in an Elderly Patient: Case Study 3**

This case involves an 80-year-old woman who presents with oral involvement and extensive skin lesions.

Diagnosis: Biopsy and clinical examination.

The treatment consists of systemic medication and topical corticosteroids, with the patient closely monitored for any adverse effects. Skincare and carer support are of utmost importance.

These examples show how a multidisciplinary team, patient education, and individualized treatment programs are crucial for controlling lichen planus in some groups.

Overall, it's important to have a detailed grasp of how lichen planus presents differently across different demographics while managing the condition in certain populations. Improving the quality of life and achieving effective management requires personalized treatment approaches, patient education, and supportive care.

CHAPTER 8

INVESTIGATIONS AND PLANS FOR THE FUTURE

Recent Developments in the Study of Lichen Planus

The skin and mucous membranes can be affected by lichen planus, an inflammatory disorder. Understanding the pathogenesis, increasing the reliability of diagnoses, and creating efficient treatments are the current directions of research. Researchers are looking into the biological mechanisms and immunological pathways that contribute to the development and progression of the disease, as well as its autoimmune nature. Environmental triggers, like stress and infections, are also being studied for their potential to worsen symptoms. More comprehensive approaches to patient care are emerging as a result of the growing body of research on the psychological and social effects of lichen planus.

Recent Advances in Immunotherapy

Immunotherapy has potential as a treatment for lichen planus, especially in cases when standard treatments have failed. One recent development is the use of biologics, which aim to suppress particular immune system components. Researchers are looking at the safety and effectiveness of drugs such as JAK inhibitors, IL-17 inhibitors, and TNF inhibitors in the treatment of lichen planus. Reducing inflammation and disease activity is the goal of these therapies, which try to modify the immune response. To find out what these new medicines can do and what risks they may have in the long run, clinical trials must be ongoing.

Innovations in Diagnostic Tools

The diagnosis of lichen planus is becoming more precise and faster as a result of technological advancements. Dermoscopy is a non-invasive imaging method that helps distinguish lichen planus from other skin disorders by providing a detailed inspection of skin lesions. The cellular features of lichen planus lesions can be better understood through histopathological examination utilizing molecular techniques and improved staining procedures. More specifically, advances in genetic testing and serological markers are allowing for earlier detection and more tailored treatment programs.

Genetic Studies and Their Results

New genetic evidence is pointing to a hereditary component of lichen planus, which may explain why some people are more likely to develop the condition than others. Several gene polymorphisms have been linked to an increased likelihood of acquiring the illness, according to studies. Additionally, novel treatment targets may be discovered by investigating the function of epigenetic alterations in lichen planus pathogenesis. Lichen planus has complex genetic components that, once understood, can aid in disease susceptibility prediction and preventative strategy customization.

New Methods of Treatment

Researchers are actively looking for new ways to cure lichen planus so that patients have better results. There is evidence that phototherapy, particularly narrowband UVB and UVA-1, can alleviate symptoms. Because of their anti-inflammatory effects, retinoids are finding usage in both topical and systemic forms. Topical treatments are becoming more effective due to advancements in drug delivery technologies like liposomes and nanoparticles, which allow the drugs to penetrate and stay in the skin longer. Herbal treatments and acupuncture are two examples of complementary and alternative medicine that are being studied for their possible advantages in lichen planus symptom management.

Taking Part in Clinical Trials

Research and treatment for lichen planus are greatly advanced by clinical trials. Their information on the effectiveness and safety of new treatments is invaluable. By taking part in clinical trials, patients not only have the chance to try new medicines, but they also help researchers better understand the disease. From new immunotherapies to dietary changes, researchers are testing a broad variety of interventions. The success of these trials depends on enrolling and retaining patients, and we are making every effort to guarantee that participants represent society at large.

How Technology Contributes to Management

Telemedicine, mobile health applications, and wearable devices are transforming the way lichen planus is managed. In underserved locations, specialized treatment can be more easily accessible through telemedicine platforms that allow for remote consultations. Tools for symptom tracking, medication adherence, and patient education are available through mobile apps. Wearable technology has the potential to track vital signs in real-time, providing doctors with actionable information. These innovations in technology allow for more precise illness monitoring, more tailored treatment programs, and better overall health results for patients.

Hopes for a Cure in the Future

The ongoing study aims to comprehend the condition at a molecular level, which bodes well for the future of lichen planus cure chances. There is hope for the development of curative medicines thanks to developments in immunotherapy, genetic studies, and regenerative medicine. To cure genetic abnormalities and fix injured tissues, scientists are investigating stem cell therapy and gene editing tools like CRISPR. Finding a solution faster requires teamwork between scientists, doctors, and pharmaceutical corporations.

Working Together and Conducting Research Across Disciplines

Improving our knowledge and ability to treat lichen planus requires teamwork and research spanning multiple disciplines. Experts from many fields are collaborating to decipher the disease's nuances, including dermatologists, immunologists, geneticists, and more. By pooling their resources and information, researchers in consortia and other forms of collaborative research can conduct more thorough and efficient studies. When it comes to financing and carrying out massive research projects, public-private partnerships are also major players. The translation of scientific discoveries into therapeutic applications relies heavily on these joint endeavors.

The Role of Patients in Scientific Investigations

Researchers looking into lichen planus can benefit from patient input in multiple ways. To help determine whether new treatments are beneficial, one of the most straightforward ways is to take part in clinical trials. Another way patients can assist researchers in understanding the disease's natural history is by participating in patient registries and observational studies.

Raising awareness and generating research money can be achieved through engaging with patient advocacy groups and sharing personal experiences. Another option is for patients to donate their biological samples to biobanks; these samples are extremely useful for genetic and molecular research. Lichen planus patients have an important impact on scientific progress and patient outcomes when they take part in research studies.

CHAPTER 9

SUPPORTING AND INSTRUCTING PATIENTS

The Value of Patient Advocates

People dealing with lichen planus must have strong patient advocates. The greatest care and support for patients can be guaranteed with the help of advocates. Greater understanding of the problem, enhanced quality of life, and more effective treatment outcomes are all possible outcomes of strong advocacy. Ensuring patients are aware of their rights and the resources that are accessible to them, empowers them to make well-informed decisions regarding their health.

Self-Advocacy Techniques

Taking an active role in your healthcare is what self-advocacy is all about. Gather as much information as you can about lichen planus, including its causes, symptoms, and available treatments. Share your thoughts and feelings with your healthcare practitioners without holding back. It is important to meticulously document your symptoms, treatments, and any adverse consequences. Do not be shy about seeking clarification or a second perspective. Your care can be greatly improved if you are aware of your rights and are not afraid to assert them.

Sharing Knowledge with Those Close to You

One way to create a supportive atmosphere for someone with lichen planus is to educate them about the condition. Be sure to include accurate information regarding the ailment, how it affects your everyday life, and how they might be of assistance. Bring them along to their doctor's appointments and support group gatherings. Misunderstandings can be lessened and your support system can be strengthened through open communication.

Programmes for Community Outreach and Education

Lichen Planus education and awareness campaigns rely heavily on community outreach programs. Health fairs, support groups, and educational seminars are all examples of programs that fall under this category. In addition to providing helpful materials, they facilitate a community where individuals may talk to one another about their struggles and get support. Being active in your community can aid in the dissemination of information, the reduction of stigma, and the pursuit of greater research and financial support for the condition.

Collaboration with Medical Professionals

You should make an effort to develop a solid rapport with your healthcare professionals. It is important to choose a healthcare specialist with expertise in lichen planus and a person you trust. Jot down any questions or concerns you may have in advance of your appointments. Tell the truth about your symptoms and how well your treatment is working. A treatment plan that is both unique and effective can be achieved via consistent communication and mutual respect.

Legal Protections and Insurance Concerns

The importance of knowing your insurance coverage and legal rights cannot be overstated. Lichen planus patients may have legal rights under disability legislation. Find out what kinds of medical care and prescription drugs are covered by reviewing your insurance policy. Think about seeing a lawyer or patient advocate if you run into problems. To get the benefits to which you are due, they can help you with appeals.

How to Find Your Way Around the Healthcare System

Navigating the healthcare system may be quite challenging and intimidating. The first step is to familiarise yourself with the various healthcare providers and services that are offered. Get the hang of managing your medical information, getting the appropriate authorizations, and navigating referrals. If you need assistance coordinating your treatment or gaining access to essential services, patient navigators or advocates are available to help.

Launching Public Education Drives

To educate both the general population and lawmakers about lichen planus, awareness campaigns are crucial. Get the word out through a variety of channels, including social media, community events, and collaborations with other groups. Bring attention to real-life patient experiences, disseminate findings from scientific studies, and push for more research and funding. Campaigns that succeed in raising lichen planus awareness can help people better understand the condition and rally behind individuals who suffer from it.

Collaboration with Groups Focused on Lichen Planus

You can get more help and resources if you work with groups that are specifically for lichen planus. Among the many services provided by these groups are advocacy opportunities, support groups, and educational resources. You can get in touch with researchers, community events, and specialists with their assistance. Collaborating with these organizations enhances our combined endeavor to enhance patient outcomes and increase consciousness.

Tools for Continual Education

To find out more about lichen planus, you can use any number of resources. There is a plethora of information available through credible websites, medical publications, and patient groups. For a sense of community, think about signing up for a support group or participating in an online forum. If you want to take charge of your health and the health of others around you, staying informed is key.

Individuals with lichen planus can better manage their illness and increase their chances of receiving optimal care and support if they learn about and practice these components of patient advocacy and education.

CHAPTER 10

ANSWERS TO COMMON QUESTIONS

Misconceptions Regarding Lichen Planus

One common misconception is that lichen planus can spread from person to person.

Spread of lichen planus is not possible. The cause of this inflammatory illness is unclear, although it is thought to be associated with an immune system issue.

Second Myth: Lichen Planus Only Affects Adults.

Although Lichen Planus is more prevalent in middle-aged people, it can also affect children and teenagers.

Myth 3: The skin is always impacted by Lichen Planus.

An infection of the skin, mucous membranes, nails, or hair can be caused by lichen planus. Additionally common is oral lichen planus, which affects the inner surface of the mouth.

Myth #4: Lichen Planus may be cured.

There may not be a cure for lichen planus just yet, but there are plenty of ways to alleviate the symptoms.

1. **Skin Care:** To lessen redness and irritation, use mild, fragrance-free cleansers and moisturizers.

2. **Avoid Triggers:** Figure out what could set you off, including stress, specific drugs, or allergies, and stay away from them.

3. If your doctor has recommended corticosteroids or retinoids, be sure to take them exactly as directed.

4. Good dental hygiene and the use of prescribed mouthwashes can help alleviate oral lichen planus.

5. Visit your dermatologist or primary care physician for checkups regularly to keep an eye on the problem.

Dealing with Difficult Situations and Emergencies

Please contact your healthcare practitioner without delay in the event of a serious flare-up. Alternative treatments or harsher medicines may be recommended.

Infections are a potential complication of lichen planus lesions. Redness, heat, swelling, and pus are all symptoms of an infection. Make an immediate appointment with a doctor.

To alleviate severe pain caused by oral lichen planus, systemic therapies or specialized mouthwashes may be necessary.

When Planning a Trip

1. Take all of your prescribed medications with you on your trip, and bring extra in case any of them become delayed.

2. Keep a brief synopsis of your medical history and any medications you are taking on hand in case you get sick or hurt and need to see a doctor.

3. Wearing a hat, high-SPF sunscreen, and other sun protection measures will help keep your skin safe from the sun's harmful rays.

4. **Health:** Even when traveling, make sure to keep up with your regular skin and oral hygiene practices.

Problems That People Often Face

Medications or over-the-counter antihistamines can be used to manage itching.

-       **Exploration:**   Post-healing hyperpigmentation or dark patches may be visible. For cosmetic procedures, it's best to contact a dermatologist and use mild skincare products.

Avoid using harsh, drying cosmetics, and make sure your skin is well-moisturized to prevent dryness.

1. **Soft-Brush Technique:** Apply toothpaste that is mild and a toothbrush with soft bristles.

2. **Avoid Irritants:** Keep away from meals that can irritate oral lesions, such as spicy, acidic, or abrasive foods.

3. For the best management of oral lichen planus, it is recommended that you visit your dentist regularly.

4. To manage pain, use the prescribed mouth rinses or apply topical remedies.

Emotional Health and Stress Reduction

- **Methods for Reducing Stress**: Make time to practice relaxation techniques like yoga, deep breathing, or meditation.

- **Counselling:** If you are depressed or anxious about your condition, it may be helpful to contact a therapist or counselor.

- Enrol in a support group where you can talk to people who understand what it's like to live with lichen planus and get advice on how to deal with the condition.

What to Eat

Include anti-inflammatory foods in your diet, like fruits, vegetables, and omega-3 fatty acids.

- **Avoid Triggers:** Keep out Acidic and Spicy Foods: If you suffer from Oral Lichen Planus, it's important to know which foods make your symptoms worse and to avoid them.

- **Healthy Eating:** Eat a variety of foods to keep your body and immune system in good working order.

Resources for Obtaining Help

Support Groups: Seek out groups that cater to people living with lichen planus, either in your area or online.

Healthcare Providers: Seek advice from specialists including your primary care physician, dentist, and dermatologist as needed.

- **Resources for Education:** When seeking knowledge, use authoritative organizations like the NIH or the American Academy of Dermatology.

Closing Remarks of Support and Guidance

You can live a fulfilling life with Lichen Planus with the right management and support. Respect your doctor's orders, learn as much as you can about your illness, and ask for help when you need it. Always keep in mind that there are several tools available to assist you in efficiently managing your health and well-being and that you are not facing this path alone.

www.ingramcontent.com/pod-product-compliance
Lightning Source LLC
Chambersburg PA
CBHW061250250726
48653CB00002B/601